Simple Keto Chaffle Cookbook

50 Easy and Tasty Chaffle Recipes

Imogene Cook

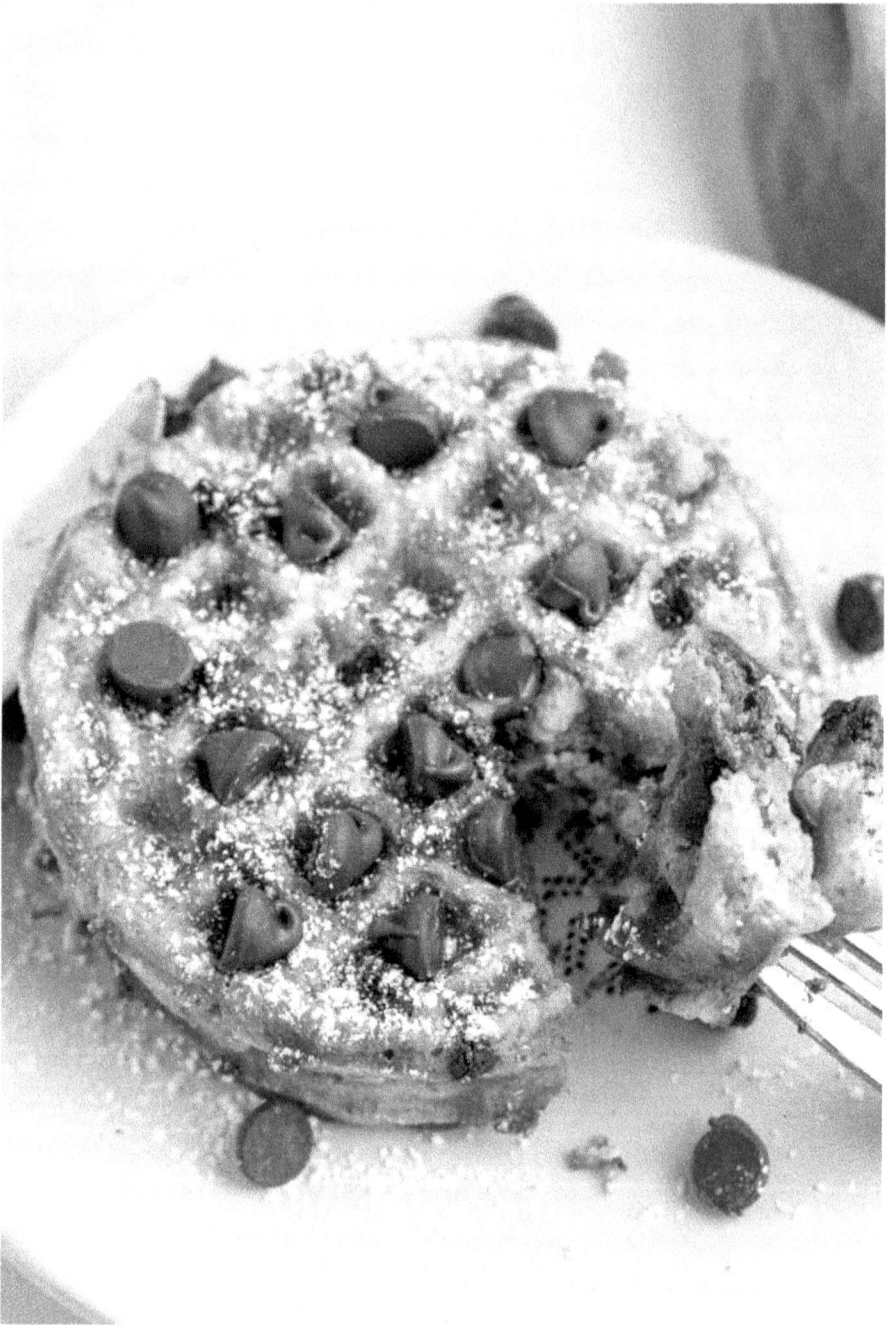

TABLE OF CONTENTS

How to Make Chaffles?

Equipment and Ingredients Discussed

Making chaffles requires five simple steps and nothing more than a waffle maker for flat chaffles and a waffle bowl maker for chaffle bowls.

To make chaffles, you will need two necessary ingredients –eggs and cheese. My preferred cheeses are cheddar cheese or mozzarella cheese. These melt quickly, making them the go-to for most recipes. Meanwhile, always ensure that your cheeses are finely grated or thinly sliced for use.

Now, to make a standard chaffle:

First, preheat your waffle maker until adequately hot.

Meanwhile, in a bowl, mix the egg with cheese on hand until well combined.

Open the iron, pour in a quarter or half of the mixture, and close.

Cook the chaffle for 5 to 7 minutes or until it is crispy.

Transfer the chaffle to a plate and allow cooling before serving.

11 Tips to Make Chaffles

My surefire ways to turn out the crispiest of chaffles:

Preheat Well: Yes! It sounds obvious to preheat the waffle iron before usage. However, preheating the iron moderately

will not get your chaffles as crispy as you will like. The best way to preheat before cooking is to ensure that the iron is very hot.

Not-So-Cheesy: Will you prefer to have your chaffles less cheesy? Then use mozzarella cheese.

Not-So Eggy: If you aren't comfortable with the smell of eggs in your chaffles, try using egg whites instead of egg yolks or whole eggs.

To Shred or to Slice: Many recipes call for shredded cheese when making chaffles, but I find sliced cheeses to offer crispier pieces. While I stick with mostly shredded cheese for convenience's sake, be at ease to use sliced cheese in the same quantity. When using sliced cheeses, arrange two to four pieces in the waffle iron, top with the beaten eggs, and some slices of the cheese. Cover and cook until crispy.

Shallower Irons: For better crisps on your chaffles, use shallower waffle irons as they cook easier and faster.

Layering: Don't fill up the waffle iron with too much batter. Work between a quarter and a half cup of total ingredients per batch for correctly done chaffles.

Patience: It is a virtue even when making chaffles. For the best results, allow the chaffles to sit in the iron for 5 to 7 minutes before serving.

No Peeking: 7 minutes isn't too much of a time to wait for the outcome of your chaffles, in my opinion.

Opening the iron and checking on the chaffle before

it is done stands you a worse chance of ruining it.

Crispy Cooling: For better crisp, I find that allowing the chaffles to cool further after they are transferred to a plate aids a lot.

Easy Cleaning: For the best cleanup, wet a paper towel and wipe the inner parts of the iron clean while still warm. Kindly note that the iron should be warm but not hot!

Brush It: Also, use a clean toothbrush to clean between the iron's teeth for a thorough cleanup. You may also use a dry, rough sponge to clean the iron while it is still warm.

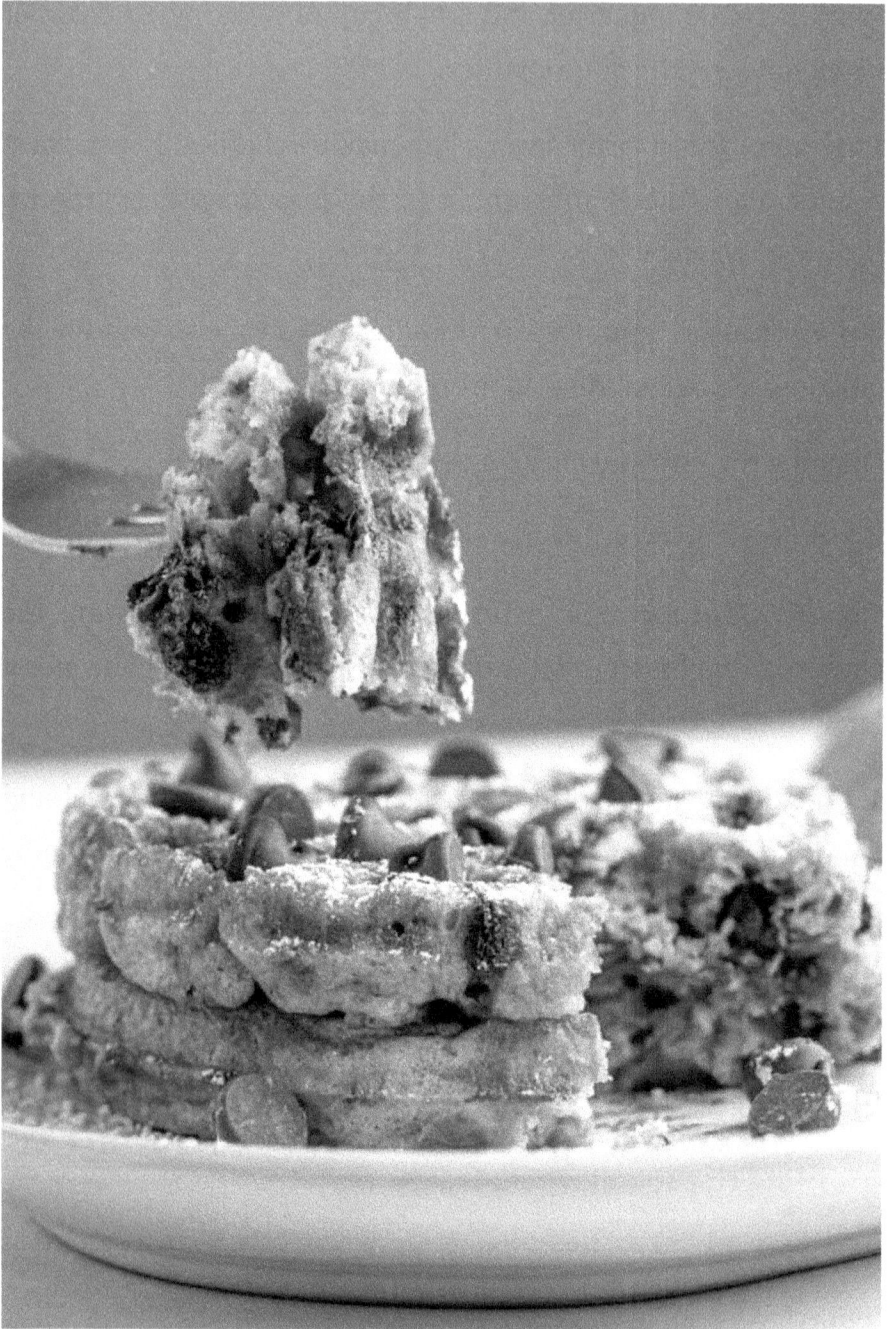

Layered Cheese Chaffles

Preparation time: 8 minutes

Cooking Time: 5 Minutes

Servings: 2

Ingredients:

- 1 organic egg, beaten
- 1/3 cup Cheddar cheese, shredded
- ½ teaspoon ground flaxseed
- ¼ teaspoon organic baking powder
- 2 tablespoons Parmesan cheese, shredded

Directions:

1. Preheat a mini waffle iron and then grease it.
2. In a bowl, place all the ingredients except Parmesan and beat until well combined.
3. Place half the Parmesan cheese in the bottom of preheated waffle iron.
4. Place half of the egg mixture over cheese and top with the remaining Parmesan cheese.
5. Cook for about 3-minutes or until golden brown.

6. Serve warm.

Nutrition:

Calories:264 Net Carb:1 Fat:20g Saturated Fat:11.1g Carbohydrate:2.1g Dietary Fiber:0.4g Sugar:0.6g Protein:18.9g

Chaffles With Keto Ice Cream

Preparation time: 10 minutes

Cooking Time: 14 Minutes

Servings: 2

Ingredients:

- 1 egg, beaten
- ½ cup finely grated mozzarella cheese
- ¼ cup almond flour
- 2 tbsp swerve confectioner's sugar
- 1/8 tsp xanthan gum
- Low-carb ice cream (flavor of your choice) for serving

Directions:

1. Preheat the waffle iron.
2. In a medium bowl, mix all the ingredients except the ice cream.
3. Open the iron and add half of the mixture. Close and cook until crispy, 7 minutes.
4. Transfer the chaffle to a plate and make second one with the remaining batter.

5. On each chaffle, add a scoop of low carb ice cream, fold into half-moons and enjoy.

Nutrition:

Calories 89 Fats 48g Carbs 1.67g Net Carbs 1.37g Protein 5.91g

Vanilla Mozzarella Chaffles

Preparation time: 10 minutes

Cooking Time: 12 Minutes

Servings: 2

Ingredients:

- 1 organic egg, beaten
- 1 teaspoon organic vanilla extract
- 1 tablespoon almond flour
- 1 teaspoon organic baking powder
- Pinch of ground cinnamon
- 1 cup Mozzarella cheese, shredded

Directions:

1. Preheat a mini waffle iron and then grease it.
2. In a bowl, place the egg and vanilla extract and beat until well combined.
3. Add the flour, baking powder and cinnamon and mix well.
4. Add the Mozzarella cheese and stir to combine.

5. In a small bowl, place the egg and Mozzarella cheese and stir to combine.

6. Place half of the mixture into preheated waffle iron and cook for about 5-minutes or until golden brown.

7. Repeat with the remaining mixture.

8. Serve warm.

Nutrition:

Calories:103 Net Carb:2.4g Fat:6.6g Saturated Fat:2.3g Carbohydrates: 2. Dietary Fiber: 0.5g Sugar: 0.6g Protein: 6.8g

Bruschetta Chaffle

Preparation time: 10 minutes

Cooking Time: 5 Minutes

Servings: 2

Ingredients:

- 2 basic chaffles
- 2 tablespoons sugar-free marinara sauce
- 2 tablespoons mozzarella, shredded
- 1 tablespoon olives, sliced
- 1 tomato sliced
- 1 tablespoon keto friendly pesto sauce
- Basil leaves

Directions:

1. Spread marinara sauce on each chaffle.
2. Spoon pesto and spread on top of the marinara sauce.
3. Top with the tomato, olives and mozzarella.
4. Bake in the oven for 3 minutes or until the cheese has melted.
5. Garnish with basil.

6. Serve and enjoy.

Nutrition:

Calories 182 Total Fat 11g Saturated Fat 6.1g Cholesterol 30mg Sodium 508mg Potassium 1mg Total Carbohydrate 3.1g Dietary Fiber 1.1g Protein 16.8g Total Sugars 1g

Egg-free Psyllium Husk Chaffles

Preparation time: 8 minutes

Cooking Time: 4 Minutes

Servings: 3

Ingredients:

- 1 ounce Mozzarella cheese, shredded
- 1 tablespoon cream cheese, softened
- 1 tablespoon psyllium husk powder

Directions:

1. Preheat a waffle iron and then grease it.
2. In a blender, place all ingredients and pulse until a slightly crumbly mixture forms.
3. Place the mixture into preheated waffle iron and cook for about 4 minutes or until golden brown.
4. Serve warm.

Nutrition:

Calories:137 Net Carb:1.3g Fat:8.8g Saturated Fat:2g Carbohydrates: 1.3g Dietary Fiber: 0g Sugar: 0g Protein: 9.5g

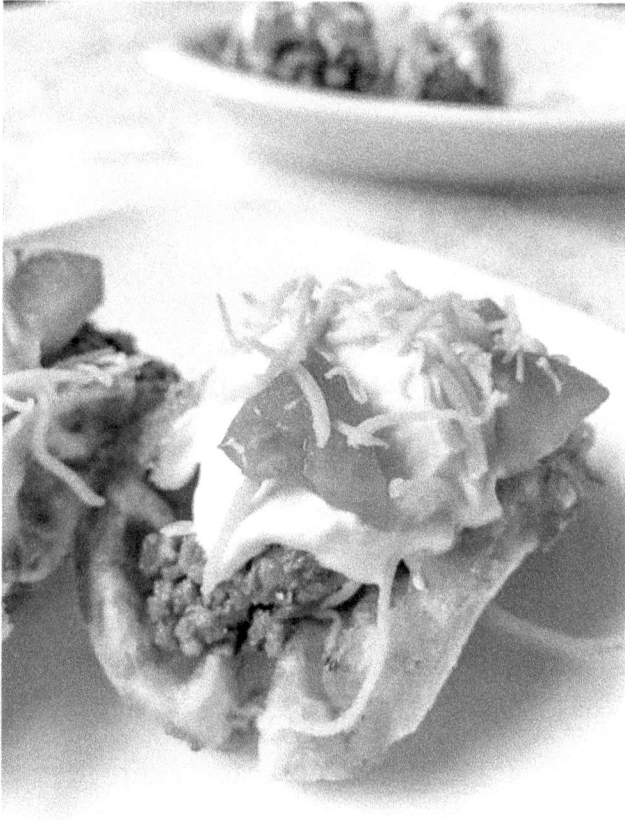

Mozzarella & Almond Flour Chaffles

Preparation time: 10 minutes

Cooking Time: 8 Minutes

Servings: 4

Ingredients:

- ½ cup Mozzarella cheese, shredded
- 1 large organic egg
- 2 tablespoons blanched almond flour
- ¼ teaspoon organic baking powder

Directions:

1. Preheat a mini waffle iron and then grease it.
2. In a medium bowl, place all ingredients and with a fork, mix until well combined.
3. Place half of the mixture into preheated waffle iron and cook for about 4 minutes or until golden brown.
4. Repeat with the remaining mixture.
5. Serve warm.

Nutrition:

Calories: 98 Net Carb: 1.4g Fat: 7.1g Saturated Fat: 1g

Carbohydrates: 2.2g Dietary Fiber: 0.8g Sugar: 0.2g Protein: 7g

Pulled Pork Chaffle Sandwiches

Preparation time: 9 minutes

Cooking Time: 28 Minutes

Servings: 2

Ingredients:

- 2 eggs, beaten
- 1 cup finely grated cheddar cheese
- ¼ tsp baking powder
- 2 cups cooked and shredded pork
- 1 tbsp sugar-free BBQ sauce
- 2 cups shredded coleslaw mix
- 2 tbsp apple cider vinegar
- ½ tsp salt
- ¼ cup ranch dressing

Directions:

1. Preheat the waffle iron.
2. In a medium bowl, mix the eggs, cheddar cheese, and baking powder.

3. Open the iron and add a quarter of the mixture. Close and cook until crispy, 7 minutes.
4. Transfer the chaffle to a plate and make 3 more chaffles in the same manner.
5. Meanwhile, in another medium bowl, mix the pulled pork with the BBQ sauce until well combined. Set aside.
6. Also, mix the coleslaw mix, apple cider vinegar, salt, and ranch dressing in another medium bowl.
7. When the chaffles are ready, on two pieces, divide the pork and then top with the ranch coleslaw. Cover with the remaining chaffles and insert mini skewers to secure the sandwiches.
8. Enjoy afterward.

Nutrition:

Calories 374 Fats 23.61g Carbs 8.2g Net Carbs 8.2g Protein 28.05g

Cheddar & Egg White Chaffles

Preparation time: 9 minutes

Cooking Time: 12 Minutes

Servings: 2

Ingredients:

- 2 egg whites
- 1 cup Cheddar cheese, shredded

Directions:

1. Preheat a mini waffle iron and then grease it.
2. In a small bowl, place the egg whites and cheese and stir to combine.
3. Place ¼ of the mixture into preheated waffle iron and cook for about 4 minutes or until golden brown.
4. Repeat with the remaining mixture.
5. Serve warm.

Nutrition:

Calories:122   NetCarb:0.5g   Fat:9.4g   Saturated   Fat:
Carbohydrates: 0.5g Dietary Fiber: 0g Sugar: 0.3g Protein: 8.8g

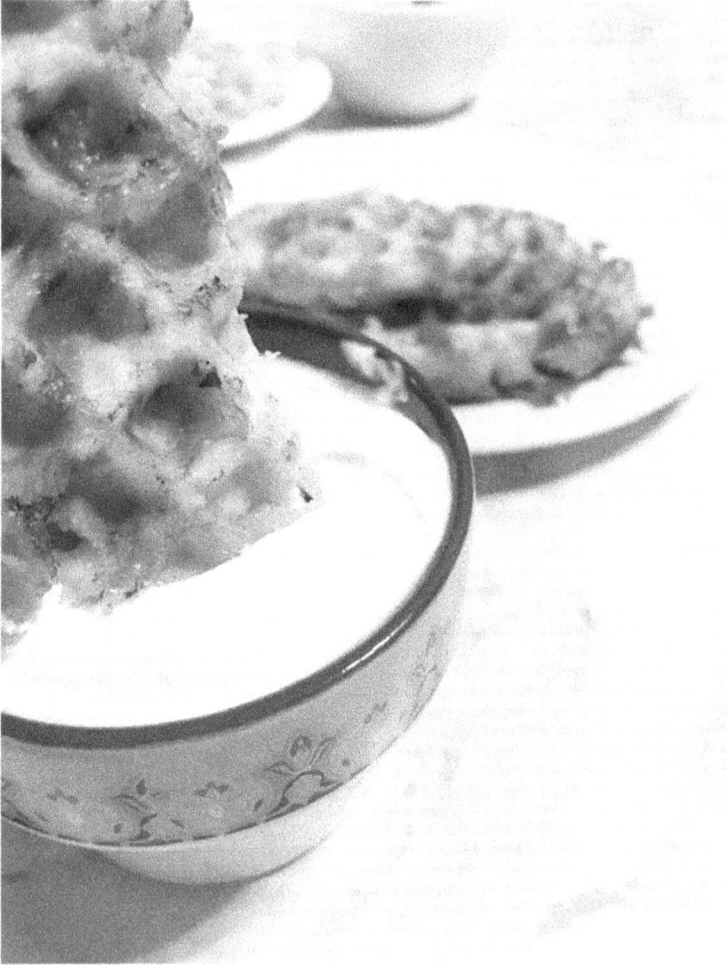

Spicy Shrimp and Chaffles

Preparation time: 9 minutes

Cooking Time: 31 Minutes

Servings: 4

Ingredients:

For the shrimp:

- 1 tbsp olive oil
- 1 lb jumbo shrimp, peeled and deveined
- 1 tbsp Creole seasoning
- Salt to taste
- 2 tbsp hot sauce
- 3 tbsp butter
- 2 tbsp chopped fresh scallions to garnish

For the chaffles:

- 2 eggs, beaten
- 1 cup finely grated Monterey Jack cheese

Directions:

For the shrimp:

1. Heat the olive oil in a medium skillet over medium heat.

2. Season the shrimp with the Creole seasoning and salt. Cook in the oil until pink and opaque on both sides, 2 minutes.
3. Pour in the hot sauce and butter. Mix well until the shrimp is adequately coated in the sauce, 1 minute.
4. Turn the heat off and set aside.

For the chaffles:

5. Preheat the waffle iron.
6. In a medium bowl, mix the eggs and Monterey Jack cheese.
7. Open the iron and add a quarter of the mixture. Close and cook until crispy, 7 minutes.
8. Transfer the chaffle to a plate and make 3 more chaffles in the same manner.
9. Cut the chaffles into quarters and place on a
10. plate.
11. Top with the shrimp and garnish with the
12. scallions.
13. Serve warm.

Nutrition:

Calories 342 Fats 19.75g Carbs 2.8g Net Carbs 2.3g Protein 36.01g

Creamy Chicken Chaffle Sandwich

Preparation time: 10 minutes

Cooking Time: 10 Minutes

Servings:2

Ingredients:

- Cooking spray
- 1 cup chicken breast fillet, cubed
- Salt and pepper to taste
- ¼ cup all-purpose cream
- 4 garlic chaffles
- Parsley, chopped

Directions:

1. Spray your pan with oil.
2. Put it over medium heat.
3. Add the chicken fillet cubes.
4. Season with salt and pepper.
5. Reduce heat and add the cream.

6. Spread chicken mixture on top of the chaffle.

7. Garnish with parsley and top with another chaffle.

Nutrition:

Calories 273 Total Fat 34g Saturated Fat 4.1g Cholesterol 62mg Sodium 373mg Total Carbohydrate 22.5g Dietary Fiber 1.1g Total Sugars 3.2g Protein 17.5g Potassium 177mg

Chaffle Cannoli

Preparation time: 9 minutes

Cooking Time: 28 Minutes

Servings: 2

Ingredients:

For the chaffles:

- 1 large egg
- 1 egg yolk
- 3 tbsp butter, melted
- 1 tbso swerve confectioner's
- 1 cup finely grated Parmesan cheese
- 2 tbsp finely grated mozzarella cheese

For the cannoli filling:

- ½ cup ricotta cheese
- 2 tbsp swerve confectioner's sugar
- 1 tsp vanilla extract
- 2 tbsp unsweetened chocolate chips for garnishing

Directions:

1. Preheat the waffle iron.
2. Meanwhile, in a medium bowl, mix all the ingredients for the chaffles.
3. Open the iron, pour in a quarter of the mixture, cover, and cook until crispy, 7 minutes.
4. Remove the chaffle onto a plate and make 3 more with the remaining batter.
5. Meanwhile, for the cannoli filling:
6. Beat the ricotta cheese and swerve confectioner's sugar until smooth. Mix in the vanilla.
7. On each chaffle, spread some of the filling and wrap over.
8. Garnish the creamy ends with some chocolate chips.
9. Serve immediately.

Nutrition:

Calories 308 Fats 25.05g Carbs 5.17g Net Carbs 5.17g Protein 15.18g

Strawberry Shortcake Chaffle Bowls

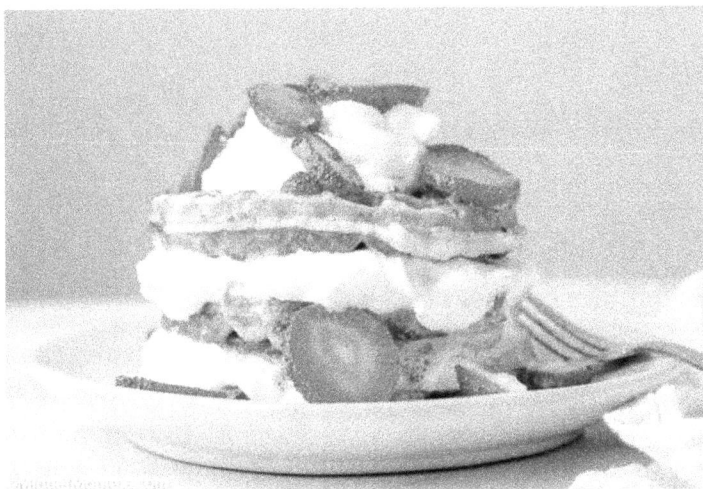

Preparation time: 15 minutes

Cooking Time: 28 Minutes

Servings: 2

Ingredients:

- 1 egg, beaten
- ½ cup finely grated mozzarella cheese
- 1 tbsp almond flour
- ¼ tsp baking powder
- 2 drops cake batter extract
- 1 cup cream cheese, softened

- 1 cup fresh strawberries, sliced
- 1 tbsp sugar-free maple syrup

Directions:

1. Preheat a waffle bowl maker and grease lightly with cooking spray.
2. Meanwhile, in a medium bowl, whisk all the ingredients except the cream cheese and strawberries.
3. Open the iron, pour in half of the mixture, cover, and cook until crispy, 6 to 7 minutes.
4. Remove the chaffle bowl onto a plate and set aside.
5. Make a second chaffle bowl with the remaining batter.
6. To serve, divide the cream cheese into the chaffle bowls and top with the strawberries.
7. Drizzle the filling with the maple syrup and serve.

Nutrition:

Calories 235 Fats 20.62g Carbs 5.9g Net Carbs 5g Protein 7.51g

Chocolate Melt Chaffles

Preparation time: 9 minutes

Cooking Time: 36 Minutes

Servings: 2

Ingredients:

For the chaffles:

- 2 eggs, beaten
- ¼ cup finely grated Gruyere cheese
- 2 tbsp heavy cream
- 1 tbsp coconut flour
- 2 tbsp cream cheese, softened
- 3 tbsp unsweetened cocoa powder
- 2 tsp vanilla extract
- A pinch of salt

For the chocolate sauce:

- 1/3 cup + 1 tbsp heavy cream
- 1 ½ oz unsweetened baking chocolate, chopped
- 1 ½ tsp sugar-free maple syrup
- 1 ½ tsp vanilla extract

Directions:

For the chaffles:

1. Preheat the waffle iron.
2. In a medium bowl, mix all the ingredients for the chaffles.
3. Open the iron and add a quarter of the mixture. Close and cook until crispy, 7 minutes.
4. Transfer the chaffle to a plate and make 3 more with the remaining batter.

For the chocolate sauce:

5. Pour the heavy cream into saucepan and simmer over low heat, 3 minutes.
6. Turn the heat off and add the chocolate. Allow melting for a few minutes and stir until fully melted, 5 minutes.
7. Mix in the maple syrup and vanilla extract.
8. Assemble the chaffles in layers with the chocolate sauce sandwiched between each layer.
9. Slice and serve immediately.

Nutrition:

Calories 172 Fats 13.57g Carbs 6.65g Net Carbs 3.65g Protein 5.76g

Pumpkin & Pecan Chaffle

Preparation time: 10 minutes

Cooking Time: 10 Minutes

Servings: 2

Ingredients:

- 1 egg, beaten
- ½ cup mozzarella cheese, grated
- ½ teaspoon pumpkin spice
- 1 tablespoon pureed pumpkin
- 2 tablespoons almond flour
- 1 teaspoon sweetener
- 2 tablespoons pecans, chopped

Directions:

1. Turn on the waffle maker.
2. Beat the egg in a bowl.
3. Stir in the rest of the ingredients.
4. Pour half of the mixture into the device.
5. Seal the lid.
6. Cook for 5 minutes.

7. Remove the chaffle carefully.

8. Repeat the steps to make the second chaffle.

Nutrition:

Calories 210 Total Fat 17 g Saturated Fat 10 g Cholesterol 110 mg Sodium 250 mg Potassium 570 mg Total Carbohydrate 4.6 g Dietary Fiber 1.7 g Protein 11 g Total Sugars 2 g

Spicy Jalapeno & Bacon Chaffles

Preparation time: 10 minutes

Servings:2

Cooking Time: 5 Minutes

Ingredients:

- 1 oz. cream cheese
- 1 large egg
- 1/2 cup cheddar cheese
- 2 tbsps. bacon bits
- 1/2 tbsp. jalapenos
- 1/4 tsp baking powder

Directions:

1. Switch on your waffle maker.
2. Grease your waffle maker with cooking spray and let it heat up.
3. Mix together egg and vanilla extract in a bowl first.
4. Add baking powder, jalapenos and bacon bites.
5. Add in cheese last and mix together.

6. Pour the chaffles batter into the maker and cook the chaffles for about 2-3 minutes

7. Once chaffles are cooked, remove from the maker.

8. Serve hot and enjoy!

Nutrition:

Protein: 24% 5kcal Fat: 70% 175 kcal Carbohydrates: 6% 15 kcal

Zucchini Parmesan Chaffles

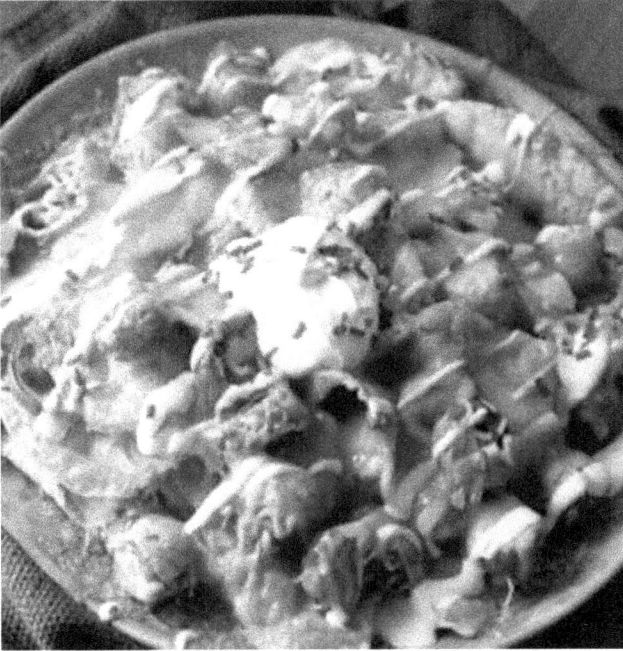

Preparation time: 10 minutes

Cooking Time: 14 Minutes

Servings: 2

Ingredients:

- 1 cup shredded zucchini
- 1 egg, beaten
- ½ cup finely grated Parmesan cheese

- Salt and freshly ground black pepper to taste

Directions:

1. Preheat the waffle iron.
2. Put all the ingredients in a medium bowl and mix well.
3. Open the iron and add half of the mixture. Close and cook until crispy, 7 minutes.
4. Remove the chaffle onto a plate and make another with the remaining mixture.
5. Cut each chaffle into wedges and serve afterward.

Nutrition:

Calories 138 Fats 9.07g Carbs 3.81g Net Carbs 3.71g Protein 10.02g

Cheddar & Almond Flour Chaffles

Preparation time: 10 minutes

Cooking Time: 10 Minutes

Servings: 2

Ingredients:

- 1 large organic egg, beaten
- ½ cup Cheddar cheese, shredded
- 2 tablespoons almond flour

Directions:

1. Preheat a mini waffle iron and then grease it.
2. In a bowl, place the egg, Cheddar cheese and almond flour and beat until well combined.
3. Place half of the mixture into preheated waffle iron and cook for about 5 minutes or until golden brown.
4. Repeat with the remaining mixture.
5. Serve warm.

Nutrition:

Calories:195 Net Carb:1g Fat:15. Saturated Fat: 7g Carbohydrates: 1.8g Dietary Fiber: 0.8g Sugar: 0.6g Protein: 10.2g

Simple& Beginner Chaffle

Preparation time: 10 minutes

Servings:2

Cooking Time: 5 Minutes

Ingredients:

- 1 large egg
- 1/2 cup mozzarella cheese, shredded
- Cooking spray

Directions:

1. Switch on your waffle maker.
2. Bcat the egg with a fork in a small mixing bowl.
3. Once the egg is beaten, add the mozzarella and mix well.
4. Spray the waffle maker with cooking spray.
5. Pour the chaffles mixture in a preheated waffle maker and let it cook for about 2-3 minutes.
6. Once the chaffles are cooked, carefully remove them from the maker and cook the remaining batter.
7. Serve hot with coffee and enjoy!

Nutrition:

Protein: 36% 42 kcal Fat: 60% 71 kcal Carbohydrates: 4% 5 kcal

Asian Cauliflower Chaffles

Preparation time: 9 minutes

Cooking Time: 28 Minutes

Servings: 2

Ingredients:

For the chaffles:

- 1 cup cauliflower rice, steamed
- 1 large egg, beaten
- Salt and freshly ground black pepper to taste 1 cup finely grated Parmesan cheese 1 tsp sesame seeds
- ¼ cup chopped fresh scallions

For the dipping sauce:

- 3 tbsp coconut aminos
- 1 ½ tbsp plain vinegar
- 1 tsp fresh ginger puree
- 1 tsp fresh garlic paste
- 3 tbsp sesame oil
- 1 tsp fish sauce
- 1 tsp red chili flakes

Directions:

1. Preheat the waffle iron.
2. In a medium bowl, mix the cauliflower rice, egg, salt, black pepper, and Parmesan cheese.
3. Open the iron and add a quarter of the mixture. Close and cook until crispy, 7 minutes.
4. Transfer the chaffle to a plate and make 3 more chaffles in the same manner.
5. Meanwhile, make the dipping sauce.
6. In a medium bowl, mix all the ingredients for the dipping sauce.
7. Plate the chaffles, garnish with the sesame seeds and scallions and serve with the dipping sauce.

Nutrition:

Calories 231 Fats 188g Carbs 6.32g Net Carbs 5.42g Protein 9.66g

Sharp Cheddar Chaffles

Preparation time: 10 minutes

Cooking Time: 10 Minutes

Servings: 2

Ingredients:

- 1 organic egg, beaten
- ½ cup sharp Cheddar cheese, shredded

Directions:

1. Preheat a mini waffle iron and then grease it.
2. In a small bowl, place the egg and cheese and stir to combine.
3. Place half of the mixture into preheated waffle iron and cook for about 5 minutes or until golden brown.
4. Repeat with the remaining mixture.
5. Serve warm.

Nutrition:

Calories: 145 Net Carb: 0.5g Fat:11. Saturated Fat:

6.6g Carbohydrates: 0.5g Dietary Fiber: 0g Sugar: 0.3g Protein: 9.8g

Egg-free Almond Flour Chaffles

Preparation time: 10 minutes

Cooking Time: 10 Minutes

Servings: 2

Ingredients:

- 2 tablespoons cream cheese, softened
- 1 cup mozzarella cheese, shredded
- 2 tablespoons almond flour
- 1 teaspoon organic baking powder

Directions:

1. Preheat a mini waffle iron and then grease it.
2. In a medium bowl, place all ingredients and with a fork, mix until well combined.
3. Place half of the mixture into preheated waffle iron and cook for about 4-5 minutes or until golden brown.
4. Repeat with the remaining mixture.
5. Serve warm.
6.

Nutrition:

Calories:77   NetCarb:2.4g   Fat:9.8g   SaturatedFat:4g Carbohydrates: 3.2g Dietary Fiber: 0.8g Sugar: 0.3g Protein: 4.8g

Mozzarellas & Psyllium Husk Chaffles

Preparation time: 10 minutes

Cooking Time: 8 Minutes

Servings: 2

Ingredients:

- ½ cup Mozzarella cheese, shredded
- 1 large organic egg, beaten
- 2 tablespoons blanched almond flour
- ½ teaspoon Psyllium husk powder
- ¼ teaspoon organic baking powder

Directions:

1. Preheat a mini waffle iron and then grease it.
2. In a bowl, place all the ingredients and beat until well combined.
3. Place half of the mixture into preheated waffle iron and cook for about 4 minutes or until golden brown.
4. Repeat with the remaining mixture.

5. Serve warm.

Nutrition:

Calories:101 Net Carb:1. Fat:7.1g Saturated Fat:1.8g Carbohydrates: 2.9g Dietary Fiber: 1.3g Sugar: 0.2g Protein: 6.7g

Pumpkin-cinnamon Churro Sticks

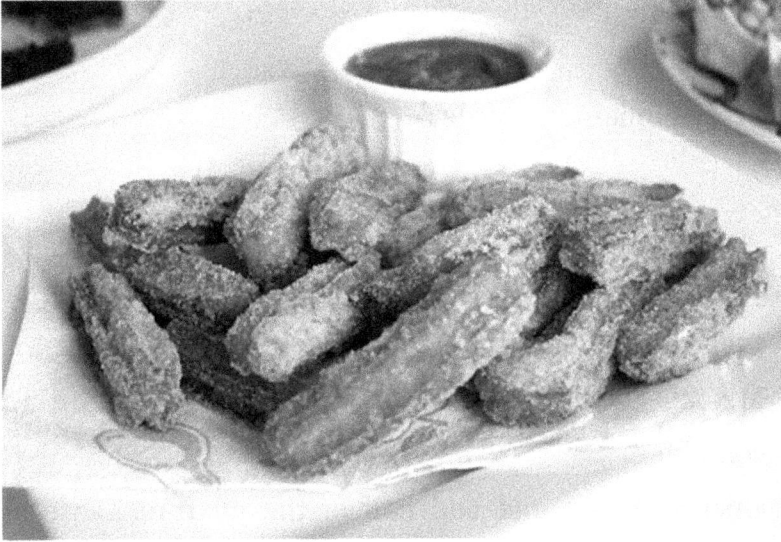

Preparation time: 10 minutes

Cooking Time: 14 Minutes

Servings: 2

Ingredients:

- 3 tbsp coconut flour
- ¼ cup pumpkin puree
- 1 egg, beaten
- ½ cup finely grated mozzarella cheese

- 2 tbsp sugar-free maple syrup + more for serving
- 1 tsp baking powder
- 1 tsp vanilla extract
- ½ tsp pumpkin spice seasoning
- 1/8 tsp salt
- 1 tbsp cinnamon powder

Directions:

1. Preheat the waffle iron.
2. Mix all the ingredients in a medium bowl until well combined.
3. Open the iron and add half of the mixture. Close and cook until golden brown and crispy, 7 minutes.
4. Remove the chaffle onto a plate and make 1 more with the remaining batter.
5. Cut each chaffle into sticks, drizzle the top with more maple syrup and serve after.

Nutrition:

Calories 219 Fats 9.72g Carbs 8.g Net Carbs 4.34g Protein 25.27g

Chicken Jalapeño Chaffles

Preparation time: 10 minutes

Cooking Time: 14 Minutes

Servings: 2

Ingredients:

- 1/8 cup finely grated Parmesan cheese
- ¼ cup finely grated cheddar cheese
- 1 egg, beaten
- ½ cup cooked chicken breasts, diced
- 1 small jalapeño pepper, deseeded and minced
- 1/8 tsp garlic powder
- 1/8 tsp onion powder
- 1 tsp cream cheese, softened

Directions:

1. Preheat the waffle iron.
2. In a medium bowl, mix all the ingredients until adequately combined.
3. Open the iron and add half of the mixture. Close and cook until crispy, 7 minutes.

4. Transfer the chaffle to a plate and make a second chaffle in the same manner.

5. Allow cooling and serve afterward.

Nutrition:

Calories 201 Fats 11.49g Carbs 3.7 Net Carbs 3.36g Protein 20.11g

Chocolate & Almond Chaffle

Preparation time: 6 minutes

Cooking Time: 12 Minutes

Servings: 2

Ingredients:

- 1 egg
- ¼ cup mozzarella cheese, shredded
- 1 oz. cream cheese
- 2 teaspoons sweetener
- 1 teaspoon vanilla
- 2 tablespoons cocoa powder
- 1 teaspoon baking powder
- 2 tablespoons almonds, chopped
- 4 tablespoons almond flour

Directions:

1. Blend all the ingredients in a bowl while the waffle maker is preheating.
2. Pour some of the mixture into the waffle maker.

3. Close and cook for 4 minutes.

4. Transfer the chaffle to a plate. Let cool for 2 minutes.

5. Repeat steps using the remaining mixture.

Nutrition:

Calories 1 Total Fat 13.1g Saturated Fat 5g Cholesterol 99mg Sodium 99mg Potassium 481mg Total Carbohydrate 9.1g Dietary Fiber 3.8g Protein 7.8g Total Sugars 0.8g

Keto Chocolate Fudge Chaffle

Preparation time: 10 minutes

Cooking Time: 14 Minutes

Servings: 2

Ingredients:

- 1 egg, beaten
- ¼ cup finely grated Gruyere cheese
- 2 tbsp unsweetened cocoa powder
- ¼ tsp baking powder
- ¼ tsp vanilla extract
- 2 tbsp erythritol
- 1 tsp almond flour
- 1 tsp heavy whipping cream
- A pinch of salt

Directions:

1. Preheat the waffle iron.
2. Add all the ingredients to a medium bowl and mix well.

3. Open the iron and add half of the mixture. Close and cook until golden brown and crispy, 7 minutes.
4. Remove the chaffle onto a plate and make another with the remaining batter.
5. Cut each chaffle into wedges and serve after.

Nutrition:

Calories 173 Fats 13.08g Carbs 3.98g Net Carbs 2.28g Protein 12.27g

Broccoli & Cheese Chaffle

Preparation time: 10 minutes

Cooking Time: 8 Minutes

Servings: 2

Ingredients:

- ¼ cup broccoli florets
- 1 egg, beaten
- 1 tablespoon almond flour
- ¼ teaspoon garlic powder
- ½ cup cheddar cheese

Directions:

1. Preheat your waffle maker.
2. Add the broccoli to the food processor.
3. Pulse until chopped.
4. Add to a bowl.
5. Stir in the egg and the rest of the ingredients.
6. Mix well.
7. Pour half of the batter to the waffle maker.

8. Cover and cook for 4 minutes.

9. Repeat procedure to make the next chaffle.

Nutrition:

Calories 170 Total Fat 13 g Saturated Fat 7 g Cholesterol 112 mg Sodium 211 mg Potassium 94 mg Total Carbohydrate 2 g Dietary Fiber 1 g Protein 11 g Total Sugars 1 g

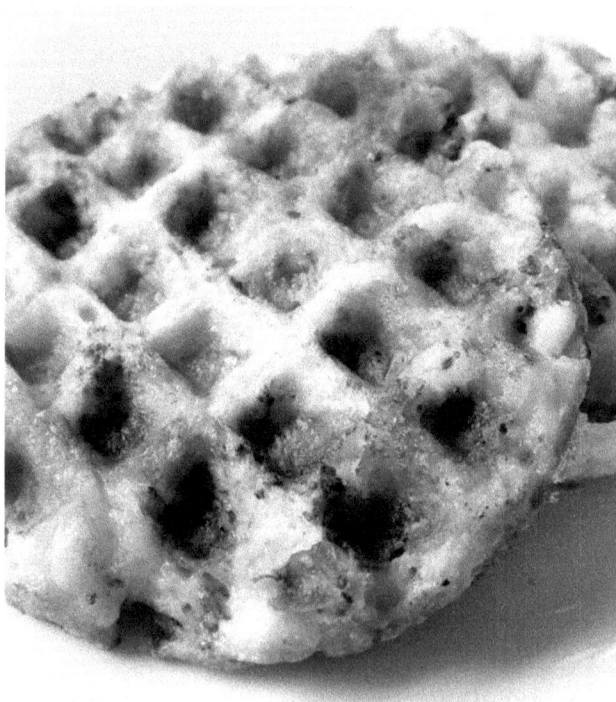

Chaffled Brownie Sundae

Preparation time: 9 minutes

Cooking Time: 30 Minutes

Servings: 2

Ingredients:

For the chaffles:

- 2 eggs, beaten
- 1 tbsp unsweetened cocoa powder
- 1 tbsp erythritol
- 1 cup finely grated mozzarella cheese

For the topping:

- 3 tbsp unsweetened chocolate, chopped
- 3 tbsp unsalted butter
- ½ cup swerve sugar
- Low-carb ice cream for topping
- 1 cup whipped cream for topping
- 3 tbsp sugar-free caramel sauce

Directions:

For the chaffles:

1. Preheat the waffle iron.
2. Meanwhile, in a medium bowl, mix all the ingredients for the chaffles.
3. Open the iron, pour in a quarter of the mixture, cover, and cook until crispy, 7 minutes.
4. Remove the chaffle onto a plate and make 3 more with the remaining batter.
5. Plate and set aside.

For the topping:

6. Meanwhile, melt the chocolate and butter in a medium saucepan with occasional stirring, 2 minutes.

To Servings:

7. Divide the chaffles into wedges and top with the ice cream, whipped cream, and swirl the chocolate sauce and caramel sauce on top.
8. Serve immediately.

Nutrition:

Calories 165 Fats 11.39g Carbs 3.81g Net Carbs 2.91g Protein 79g

Cream Cheese Chaffle

Preparation time: 10 minutes

Cooking Time: 8 Minutes

Servings: 2

Ingredients:

- 1 egg, beaten
- 1 oz. cream cheese
- ½ teaspoon vanilla
- 4 teaspoons sweetener
- ¼ teaspoon baking powder
- Cream cheese

Directions:

1. Preheat your waffle maker.
2. Add all the ingredients in a bowl.
3. Mix well.
4. Pour half of the batter into the waffle maker.
5. Seal the device.
6. Cook for 4 minutes.

7. Remove the chaffle from the waffle maker.

8. Make the second one using the same steps.

9. Spread remaining cream cheese on top before serving.

Nutrition:

Calories 169 Total Fat 14.3g Saturated Fat 7.6g Cholesterol 195mg Sodium 147mg Potassium 222mg Total Carbohydrate 4g Dietary Fiber 4g Protein 7.7g Total Sugars 0.7g

Garlic Chaffles

Preparation time: 10 minutes

Servings:4

Cooking Time: 5 Minutes

Ingredients:

- 1/2 cup mozzarella cheese, shredded
- 1/3 cup cheddar cheese
- 1 large egg
- ½ tbsp. garlic powder
- 1/2 tsp Italian seasoning
- 1/4 tsp baking powder

Directions:

1. Switch on your waffle maker and lightly grease your waffle maker with a brush.
2. Beat the egg with garlic powder, Italian seasoning and baking powder in a small mixing bowl.
3. Add mozzarella cheese and cheddar cheese to the egg mixture and mix well.

4. Pour half of the chaffles batter into the middle of your waffle iron and close the lid.
5. Cook chaffles for about 2-3 minutes Utes until crispy.
6. Once cooked, remove chaffles from the maker.
7. Sprinkle garlic powder on top and enjoy!

Nutrition:

Protein: 32% 36 kcal Fat: 61% 69 kcal Carbohydrates: 7% 7 kcal

Cinnamon Powder Chaffles

Preparation time: 10 minutes

Servings:2

Cooking Time: 5 Minutes

Ingredients:

- 1 large egg
- 3/4 cup cheddar cheese, shredded
- 2 tbsps. coconut flour
- 1/2 tbsps. coconut oil melted
- 1 tsp. stevia
- 1/2 tsp cinnamon powder
- 1/2 tsp vanilla extract
- 1/2 tsp psyllium husk powder
- 1/4 tsp baking powder

Directions:

1. Switch on your waffle maker.
2. Grease your waffle maker with cooking spray and heat up on medium heat.

3. In a mixing bowl, beat egg with coconut flour, oil, stevia, cinnamon powder, vanilla, husk powder, and baking powder.
4. Once the egg is beaten well, add in cheese and mix again.
5. Pour half of the waffle batter into the middle of your waffle iron and close the lid.
6. Cook chaffles for about 2-3 minutes Utes until crispy.
7. Once chaffles are cooked, carefully remove them from the maker.
8. Serve with keto hot chocolate and enjoy!

Nutrition:

Protein: 25% 62 kcal Fat: 72% 175 kcal Carbohydrates: 3% 7 kcal

Chaffles With Raspberry Syrup

Preparation time: 9 minutes

Cooking Time: 38 Minutes

Servings: 2

Ingredients:

For the chaffles:

- 1 egg, beaten
- ½ cup finely shredded cheddar cheese
- 1 tsp almond flour
- 1 tsp sour cream

For the raspberry syrup:

- 1 cup fresh raspberries
- ¼ cup swerve sugar
- ¼ cup water
- 1 tsp vanilla extract

Directions:

For the chaffles:

1. Preheat the waffle iron.
2. Meanwhile, in a medium bowl, mix the egg, cheddar cheese, almond flour, and sour cream.
3. Open the iron, pour in half of the mixture, cover, and cook until crispy, 7 minutes.
4. Remove the chaffle onto a plate and make another with the remaining batter.
5. For the raspberry syrup:
6. Meanwhile, add the raspberries, swerve sugar, water, and vanilla extract to a medium pot. Set over low heat and cook until the raspberries soften and sugar becomes syrupy. Occasionally stir while mashing the raspberries as you go. Turn the heat off when your desired consistency is achieved and set aside to cool.
7. Drizzle some syrup on the chaffles and enjoy when ready.

Nutrition:

Calories 105 Fats 7.11g Carbs 4.31g Net Carbs 2.21g Protein 5.83g

Egg-free Coconut Flour Chaffles

Preparation time: 10 minutes

Cooking Time: 10 Minutes

Servings: 2

Ingredients:

- 1 tablespoon flaxseed meal
- 2½ tablespoons water
- ¼ cup Mozzarella cheese, shredded
- 1 tablespoon cream cheese, softened
- 2 tablespoons coconut flour

Directions:

1. Preheat a waffle iron and then grease it.
2. In a bowl, place the flaxseed meal and water and mix well.
3. Set aside for about 5 minutes or until thickened.
4. In the bowl of flaxseed mixture, add the remaining ingredients and mix until well combined.

5. Place half of the mixture into preheated waffle iron and cook for about 3-minutes or until golden brown.
6. Repeat with the remaining mixture.
7. Serve warm.

Nutrition:

Calories:76 Net Carb:2.3g Fat:4.2g Saturated Fat:2.1g Carbohydrates: 6.3g Dietary Fiber: 4g Sugar: 0.1g Protein: 3g

Cheeseburger Chaffle

Preparation time: 10 minutes

Cooking Time: 15 Minutes

Servings: 2

Ingredients:

- 1 lb. ground beef
- 1 onion, minced
- 1 tsp. parsley, chopped
- 1 egg, beaten
- Salt and pepper to taste
- 1 tablespoon olive oil
- 4 basic chaffles
- 2 lettuce leaves
- 2 cheese slices
- 1 tablespoon dill pickles
- Ketchup
- Mayonnaise

Directions:

1. In a large bowl, combine the ground beef, onion, parsley, egg, salt and pepper.
2. Mix well.
3. Form 2 thick patties.
4. Add olive oil to the pan.
5. Place the pan over medium heat.
6. Cook the patty for 3 to 5 minutes per side or until fully cooked.
7. Place the patty on top of each chaffle.
8. Top with lettuce, cheese and pickles.
9. Squirt ketchup and mayo over the patty and veggies.
10. Top with another chaffle.

Nutrition:

Calories 325 Total Fat 16.3g Saturated Fat 6.5g Cholesterol 157mg Sodium 208mg Total Carbohydrate 3g Dietary Fiber 0.7g Total Sugars 1.4g Protein 39.6g Potassium 532mg

Buffalo Hummus Beef Chaffles

Preparation time: 9 minutes

Cooking Time: 32 Minutes

Servings: 2

Ingredients:

- 2 eggs
- 1 cup + ¼ cup finely grated cheddar cheese, divided
- 2 chopped fresh scallions
- Salt and freshly ground black pepper to taste 2 chicken breasts, cooked and diced ¼ cup buffalo sauce
- 3 tbsp low-carb hummus
- 2 celery stalks, chopped
- ¼ cup crumbled blue cheese for topping

Directions:

1. Preheat the waffle iron.
2. In a medium bowl, mix the eggs, 1 cup of the cheddar cheese, scallions, salt, and black pepper.

3. Open the iron and add a quarter of the mixture. Close and cook until crispy, 7 minutes.
4. Transfer the chaffle to a plate and make 3 more chaffles in the same manner.
5. Preheat the oven to 400 F and line a baking sheet with parchment paper. Set aside.
6. Cut the chaffles into quarters and arrange on the baking sheet.
7. In a medium bowl, mix the chicken with the buffalo sauce, hummus, and celery.
8. Spoon the chicken mixture onto each quarter of chaffles and top with the remaining cheddar cheese.
9. Place the baking sheet in the oven and bake until the cheese melts, 4 minutes.
10. Remove from the oven and top with the blue cheese.
11. Serve afterward.

Nutrition:

Calories 552 Fats 28.37g Carbs 6.97g Net Carbs 6.07g Protein 59.8g

Basic Mozzarella Chaffles

Preparation time: 10 minutes

Cooking Time: 6 Minutes

Servings: 2

Ingredients:

- 1 large organic egg, beaten
- ½ cup Mozzarella cheese, shredded finely

Directions:

1. Preheat a mini waffle iron and then grease it.
2. In a small bowl, place the egg and Mozzarella cheese and stir to combine.
3. Place half of the mixture into preheated waffle iron and cook for about 2-minutes or until golden brown.
4. Repeat with the remaining mixture.
5. Serve warm.

Nutrition:

Calories: 5 Net Carb: 0.4g Fat: 3.7g Saturated Fat: 1.5g Carbohydrates: 0.4g Dietary Fiber: 0g Sugar: 0.2g Protein: 5.2g

Brie and Blackberry Chaffles

Preparation time: 9 minutes

Cooking Time: 36 Minutes

Servings: 2

Ingredients:

For the chaffles:

- 2 eggs, beaten
- 1 cup finely grated mozzarella cheese

For the topping:

- 1 ½ cups blackberries
- 1 lemon, 1 tsp zest and 2 tbsp juice
- 1 tbsp erythritol
- 4 slices Brie cheese

Directions:

For the chaffles:

1. Preheat the waffle iron.

2. Meanwhile, in a medium bowl, mix the eggs and mozzarella cheese.

3. Open the iron, pour in a quarter of the mixture, cover, and cook until crispy, 7 minutes.

4. Remove the chaffle onto a plate and make 3 more with the remaining batter.

5. Plate and set aside.

For the topping:

6. In a medium pot, add the blackberries, lemon zest, lemon juice, and erythritol. Cook until the blackberries break and the sauce thickens, 5 minutes. Turn the heat off.

7. Arrange the chaffles on the baking sheet and place two Brie cheese slices on each. Top with blackberry mixture and transfer the baking sheet to the oven.

8. Bake until the cheese melts, 2 to 3 minutes.

9. Remove from the oven, allow cooling and serve afterward.

Nutrition:

Calories 576 Fats 42.22g Carbs 7.07g Net Carbs 3.67g Protein 42.35g

Turkey Chaffle Burger

Preparation time: 10 minutes

Cooking Time: 10 Minutes

Servings: 2

Ingredients:

- 2 cups ground turkey
- Salt and pepper to taste
- 1 tablespoon olive oil
- 4 garlic chaffles
- 1 cup Romaine lettuce, chopped
- 1 tomato, sliced
- Mayonnaise
- Ketchup

Directions:

1. Combine ground turkey, salt and pepper.
2. Form thick burger patties.
3. Add the olive oil to a pan over medium heat.
4. Cook the turkey burger until fully cooked on both sides

5. Spread mayo on the chaffle.

6. Top with the turkey burger, lettuce and tomato.

7. Squirt ketchup on top before topping with another chaffle.

Nutrition:

Calories 555 Total Fat 21.5g Saturated Fat 3.5g Cholesterol 117mg Sodium 654mg Total Carbohydrate 4.1g Dietary Fiber 2.5g Protein 31.7g Total Sugars 1g

Double Choco Chaffle

Preparation time: 10 minutes

Cooking Time: 10 Minutes

Servings: 2

Ingredients:

- 1 egg
- 2 teaspoons coconut flour
- 2 tablespoons sweetener
- 1 tablespoon cocoa powder
- ¼ teaspoon baking powder
- 1 oz. cream cheese
- ½ teaspoon vanilla
- 1 tablespoon sugar-free chocolate chips

Directions:

1. Put all the ingredients in a large bowl.
2. Mix well.
3. Pour half of the mixture into the waffle maker.
4. Seal the device.

5. Cook for 4 minutes.

6. Uncover and transfer to a plate to cool.

7. Repeat the procedure to make the second chaffle.

Nutrition:

Calories 171 Total Fat 10.7g Saturated Fat 5.3g Cholesterol 97mg

Sodium 106mg Potassium 179mg Total Carbohydrate 3g Dietary Fiber 4. Protein 5.8g Total Sugars 0.4g

Guacamole Chaffle Bites

Preparation time: 10 minutes

Cooking Time: 14 Minutes

Servings: 2

Ingredients:

- 1 large turnip, cooked and mashed
- 2 bacon slices, cooked and finely chopped
- ½ cup finely grated Monterey Jack cheese
- 1 egg, beaten
- 1 cup guacamole for topping

Directions:

1. Preheat the waffle iron.
2. Mix all the ingredients except for the guacamole in a medium bowl.
3. Open the iron and add half of the mixture. Close and cook for 4 minutes. Open the lid, flip the chaffle and cook further until golden brown and crispy, minutes.

4. Remove the chaffle onto a plate and make another in the same manner.

5. Cut each chaffle into wedges, top with the guacamole and serve afterward.

Nutrition:

Calories 311 Fats 22.52g Carbs 8.29g Net Carbs 5.79g Protein 13.g

Mayonnaise & Cream Cheese Chaffles

Preparation time: 9 minutes

Cooking Time: 20 Minutes

Servings: 2

Ingredients:

- 4 organic eggs large
- 4 tablespoons mayonnaise
- 1 tablespoon almond flour
- 2 tablespoons cream cheese, cut into small cubes

Directions:

1. Preheat a waffle iron and then grease it.
2. In a bowl, place the eggs, mayonnaise and almond flour and with a hand mixer, mix until smooth.
3. Place about ¼ of the mixture into preheated waffle iron.
4. Place about ¼ of the cream cheese cubes on top of the mixture evenly and cook for about 5 minutes or until golden brown.

5. Repeat with the remaining mixture and cream cheese cubes.

6. Serve warm.

Nutrition:

Calories: 190 Net Carb: 0.6g Fat: 17g Saturated Fat:4.2g Carbohydrates: 0.8g Dietary Fiber: 0.2g Sugar: 0.5g Protein: 6.7g

Blue Cheese Chaffle Bites

Preparation time: 10 minutes

Cooking Time: 14 Minutes

Servings: 2

Ingredients:

- 1 egg, beaten
- ½ cup finely grated Parmesan cheese
- ¼ cup crumbled blue cheese
- 1 tsp erythritol

Directions:

1. Preheat the waffle iron.
2. Mix all the ingredients in a bowl.
3. Open the iron and add half of the mixture. Close and cook until crispy, 7 minutes.
4. Remove the chaffle onto a plate and make another with the remaining mixture.
5. Cut each chaffle into wedges and serve afterward.

Nutrition:

Calories 19ats 13.91g Carbs 4.03g Net Carbs 4.03g Protein 13.48g

Raspberries Chaffles

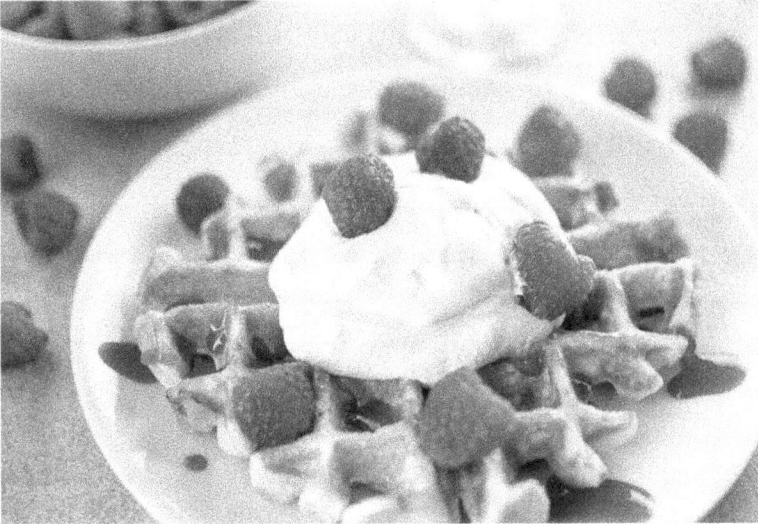

Servings:2

Cooking Time: 5 Minutes

Ingredients:

- 1 egg
- 1/2 cup mozzarella cheese, shredde
- 1 tbsp. almond flour
- 1/4 cup raspberry puree
- 1 tbsp. coconut flour for topping

Directions:

1. Preheat your waffle maker in line with the manufacturer's instructions.
2. Grease your waffle maker with cooking spray.
3. Mix together egg, almond flour, and raspberry purée.
4. Add cheese and mix until well combined.
5. Pour batter into the waffle maker.
6. Close the lid.
7. Cook for about 3-4 minutes Utes or until waffles are cooked and not soggy.
8. Once cooked, remove from the maker.
9. Sprinkle coconut flour on top and enjoy!

Nutrition:

Protein: 26% 60 kcal Fat: 63% 145 kcal Carbohydrates: 11% 25 kcal

Simple Chaffle Toast

Servings:2

Cooking Time: 5 Minutes

Ingredients:

- 1 large egg
- 1/2 cup shredded cheddar cheese

FOR TOPPING

- 1 egg
- 3-4 spinach leaves
- ¼ cup boil and shredded chicken

Directions:

1. Preheat your square waffle maker on medium-high heat.
2. Mix together egg and cheese in a bowl and make two chaffles in a chaffle maker
3. Once chaffle are cooked, carefully remove them from the maker.
4. Serve with spinach, boiled chicken, and fried egg.
5. Serve hot and enjoy!

Nutrition:

Protein: 39% 99 kcal Fat: % 153 kcal Carbohydrates: 1% 3 kcal

Savory Beef Chaffle

Preparation time: 10 minutes

Cooking Time: 15 Minutes

Servings: 2

Ingredients:

- 1 teaspoon olive oil
- 2 cups ground beef
- Garlic salt to taste
- 1 red bell pepper, sliced into strips
- 1 green bell pepper, sliced into strips
- 1 onion, minced
- 1 bay leaf
- 2 garlic chaffles
- Butter

Directions:

1. Put your pan over medium heat.
2. Add the olive oil and cook ground beef until brown.
3. Season with garlic salt and add bay leaf.

4. Drain the fat, transfer to a plate and set aside.

5. Discard the bay leaf.

6. In the same pan, cook the onion and bell peppers for 2 minutes.

7. Put the beef back to the pan.

8. Heat for 1 minute.

9. Spread butter on top of the chaffle.

10. Add the ground beef and veggies.

11. Roll or fold the chaffle.

Nutrition:

Calories 220 Total Fat 17.8g Saturated Fat 8g Cholesterol 76mg Sodium 60mg Total Carbohydrate 3g Dietary Fiber 2g Total Sugars 5.4g Protein 27.1g Potassium 537mg

Chaffles With Almond Flour

Servings:4

Cooking Time: 5 Minutes

Ingredients:

- 2 large eggs
- 1/4 cup almond flour
- 3/4 tsp baking powder
- 1 cup cheddar cheese, shredde
- Cooking spray

Directions:

1. Switch on your waffle maker and grease with cooking spray.
2. Beat eggs with almond flour and baking powder in a mixing bowl.
3. Once the eggs and cheese are mixed together, add in cheese and mix again.
4. Pour 1/cup of the batter in the dash mini waffle maker and close the lid.

5. Cook chaffles for about 2-3 minutes until crispy and cooked
6. Repeat with the remaining batter
7. Carefully transfer the chaffles to plate.
8. Serve with almonds and enjoy!

Nutrition:

Protein: 23% 52 kcal Fat: 72% 15kcal Carbohydrates: 5% 11 kcal

Nutter Butter Chaffles

Preparation time: 10 minutes

Cooking Time: 14 Minutes

Servings: 2

Ingredients:

For the chaffles:

- 2 tbsp sugar-free peanut butter powder
- 2 tbsp maple (sugar-free) syrup
- 1 egg, beaten
- ¼ cup finely grated mozzarella cheese
- ¼ tsp baking powder
- ¼ tsp almond butter
- ¼ tsp peanut butter extract
- 1 tbsp softened cream cheese

For the frosting:

- ½ cup almond flour
- 1 cup peanut butter
- 3 tbsp almond milk
- ½ tsp vanilla extract

- ½ cup maple (sugar-free) syrup

Directions:

1. Preheat the waffle iron.
2. Meanwhile, in a medium bowl, mix all the ingredients until smooth.
3. Open the iron and pour in half of the mixture.
4. Close the iron and cook until crispy, 6 to 7 minutes.
5. Remove the chaffle onto a plate and set aside.
6. Make a second chaffle with the remaining batter.
7. While the chaffles cool, make the frosting.
8. Pour the almond flour in a medium saucepan and stir-fry over medium heat until golden.
9. Transfer the almond flour to a blender and top with the remaining frosting ingredients. Process until smooth.
10. Spread the frosting on the chaffles and serve afterward.

Nutrition:

Calories 239 Fats 15.48g Carbs 17.42g Net Carbs 15.92g Protein 7.52g

Keto Reube

n Chaffles

Preparation time: 9 minutes

Cooking Time: 28 Minutes

Servings: 2

Ingredients:

For the chaffles:

- 2 eggs, beaten
- 1 cup finely grated Swiss cheese
- 2 tsp caraway seeds
- 1/8 tsp salt
- ½ tsp baking powder

For the sauce:

- 2 tbsp sugar-free ketchup
- 3 tbsp mayonnaise
- 1 tbsp dill relish
- 1 tsp hot sauce

For the filling:

- 6 oz pastrami
- 2 Swiss cheese slices
- ¼ cup pickled radishes

Directions:

For the chaffles:

1. Preheat the waffle iron.
2. In a medium bowl, mix the eggs, Swiss cheese, caraway seeds, salt, and baking powder.
3. Open the iron and add a quarter of the mixture. Close and cook until crispy, 7 minutes.
4. Transfer the chaffle to a plate and make 3 more chaffles in the same manner.

For the sauce:

5. In another bowl, mix the ketchup, mayonnaise, dill relish, and hot sauce.

To assemble:

6. Divide on two chaffles; the sauce, the pastrami, Swiss cheese slices, and pickled radishes.
7. Cover with the other chaffles, divide the sandwich in halves and serve.

Nutrition:

Calories 316 Fats 21.78g Carbs 6.52g Net Carbs 5.42g Protein 23.56g

Carrot Chaffle Cake

Servings: 6

Cooking Time: 24 Minutes

Ingredients:

- 1 egg, beaten
- 2 tablespoons melted butter
- ½ cup carrot, shredded
- ¾ cup almond flour
- 1 teaspoon baking powder
- 2 tablespoons heavy whipping cream
- 2 tablespoons sweetener
- 1 tablespoon walnuts, chopped
- 1 teaspoon pumpkin spice
- 2 teaspoons cinnamon

Directions:

1. Preheat your waffle maker.
2. In a large bowl, combine all the ingredients.
3. Pour some of the mixture into the waffle maker.
4. Close and cook for minutes.

5. Repeat steps until all the remaining batter has been used.

Nutrition:

Calories 294 Total Fat 27g Saturated Fat 12g Cholesterol 133mg Sodium 144mg Potassium 421mg Total Carbohydrate 11.6g Dietary Fiber 4.5g Protein 6.8g Total Sugars 1.7g

Cheese Slices Chaffles

Preparation time: 8 minutes

Cooking Time: 6 Minutes

Servings: 2

Ingredients:

- 2 ounces Colby Jack cheese, cut into thin triangle slices
- 1 large organic egg, beaten

Directions:

1. Preheat a waffle iron and then grease it.
2. Arrange 1 thin layer of cheese slices in the bottom of preheated waffle iron.
3. Place the beaten egg on top of the cheese.
4. Now, arrange another layer of cheese slices on top to cover evenly.
5. Cook for about 6 minutes or until golden brown.
6. Serve warm.

Nutrition:

Calories:292   NetCarb:2.4g   Fat:23g   Saturated   Fat:13.6g
Carbohydrates: 2.4g Dietary Fiber: 0g Sugar: 0.4g Protein:
18.3g

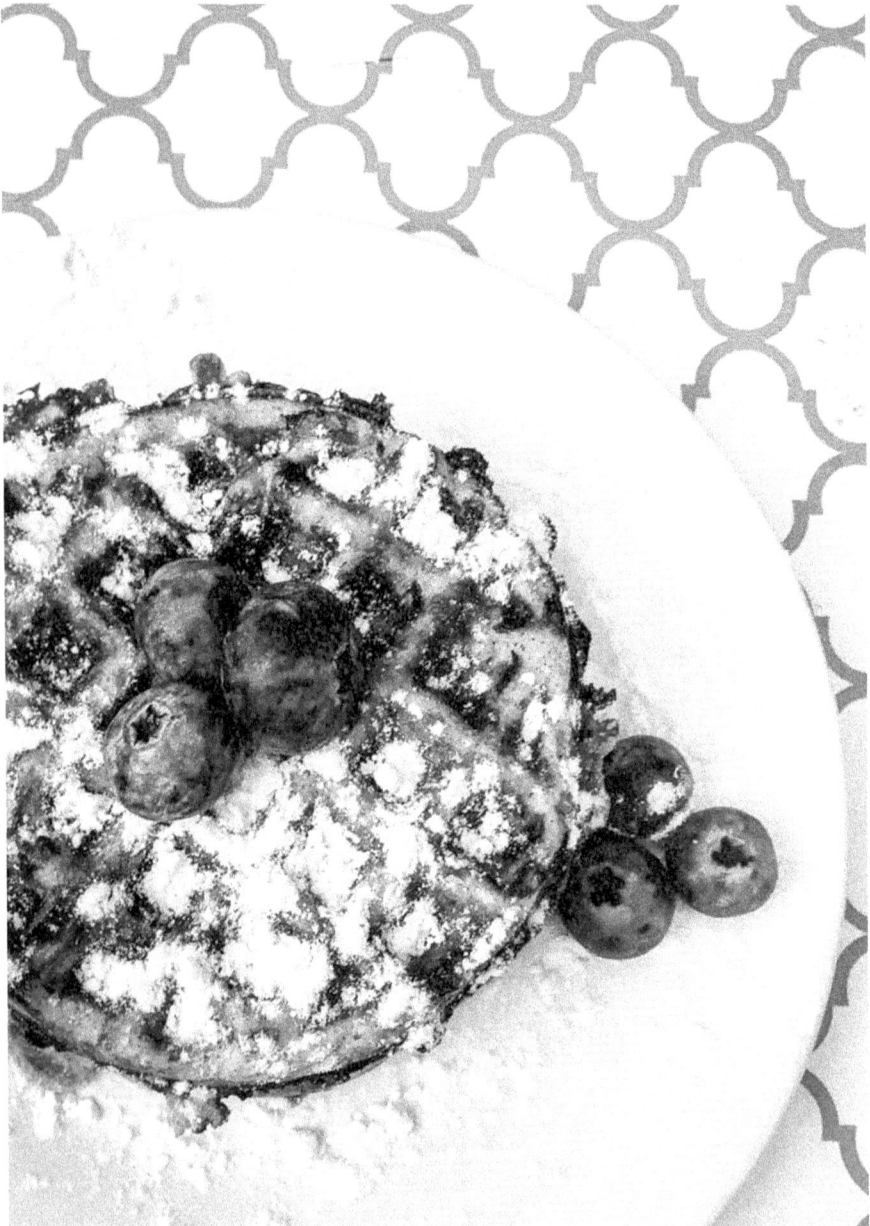

www.ingramcontent.com/pod-product-compliance
Lightning Source LLC
Chambersburg PA
CBHW050759030426
42336CB00012B/1876